OSTEOPOROSIS

A Major Concern for Older Adults

Comprehensive Guide to Preventing and Managing Osteoporosis, Bone Density Loss, and Fractures with Diet, Exercise, and Medical Treatments

Cormac Cristiano

Copyright © 2024 by Cormac Cristiano

All rights reserved. No part of this publication may be reproduced, distributed, or transmitted in any form or by any means, including photocopying, recording, or other electronic or mechanical methods, without the prior written permission of the publisher, except in the case of brief quotations embodied in critical reviews and certain other noncommercial uses permitted by copyright law.

Published by: Cormac Cristiano

Disclaimer

This book, *Osteoporosis – A Major Concern for Older Adults: Comprehensive Guide to Preventing and Managing Osteoporosis, Bone Density Loss, and Fractures with Diet, Exercise, and Medical Treatments*, is intended for informational purposes only. The information presented in this book is not a substitute for professional medical advice, diagnosis, or treatment. Always seek the advice of your physician or other qualified health providers with any questions you may have regarding a medical condition, including osteoporosis and related health issues. Never disregard professional medical advice or delay seeking it because of something you have read in this book.

The author and publisher make no representations or warranties concerning the accuracy, applicability, fitness, or completeness of the contents of this book. The information provided is based on the author's research, understanding, and experiences at the time of publication and may be subject to change as new research and information become available. The reader assumes full responsibility for any decisions made based on the information presented in this book.

The author and publisher disclaim any liability for any direct, indirect, or incidental loss or damage incurred by following the recommendations or relying on the information in this book.

Furthermore, the author does not endorse or promote any specific individuals, products, websites, organizations, or any other entities that may be referenced in this book. Any mention of such names, products, or organizations is intended solely to provide information to readers.

About This Book

Osteoporosis – A Major Concern for Older Adults: Comprehensive Guide to Preventing and Managing Osteoporosis, Bone Density Loss, and Fractures with Diet, Exercise, and Medical Treatments" provides essential insights into a condition that significantly affects older adults worldwide. The book begins with an in-depth understanding of osteoporosis, explaining its causes, the biological process of bone loss, and why early detection is critical. It emphasizes how this condition impacts quality of life, leading to fractures and long-term complications.

The book highlights the importance of bone density and educates readers on how understanding this concept is central to managing and preventing the progression of osteoporosis. The book positions osteoporosis as a major health concern that requires lifelong management, making it relevant not just to those diagnosed but to all older adults at risk.

The guide underscores the importance of prevention, drawing attention to how a proactive approach is key to long-term bone health. It discusses the biological changes in bones as people age and explores preventive strategies such as diet, exercise, and medications, making it clear that prevention must be a priority throughout one's life. The role of healthcare professionals is also covered, guiding readers on how medical support can contribute to a successful preventive plan.

The detailed coverage on the structure and function of bones, along with the bone remodeling process, provides clarity on how bones maintain strength and the importance of reaching peak bone mass in early adulthood. Readers will appreciate the explanations on the vital roles of calcium, Vitamin D, and other nutrients that are necessary for maintaining bone density, as well as the factors like hormones and lifestyle choices that affect bone health.

The book offers a thorough exploration of risk factors for osteoporosis, helping readers identify potential threats to their bone health early on. It addresses the significant impacts of age, hormonal changes, and medical conditions, while also recognizing how lifestyle choices such as diet, physical activity, and even alcohol and smoking habits can drastically influence bone health.

A comprehensive section on essential nutrients helps readers understand the critical role that proper nutrition plays in maintaining strong bones. From calcium and Vitamin D to magnesium and Vitamin K, the book provides practical advice on how to ensure your diet supports bone health. Additionally, it offers insights into how hydration, protein intake, and even minimizing caffeine and salt can help improve bone density. For those considering supplements, the book provides guidance on when and how to use them to enhance bone strength.

The exercise section provides valuable guidance on the types of physical activities most beneficial for bone health. Weight-bearing exercises, strength training, and flexibility routines are highlighted as key strategies for maintaining bone density, especially for those already diagnosed with osteoporosis.

The importance of balancing exercises to prevent falls is emphasized, as falling poses a major risk to individuals with weakened bones. By offering clear, realistic exercise goals and addressing the needs of beginners, the book ensures that all readers can take positive steps toward improving their bone health through physical activity.

A key feature of this guide is its in-depth exploration of medical treatments and medications. The book provides an overview of available medications, explaining how treatments like bisphosphonates, hormone therapies, and calcium supplements work to slow down bone loss and increase bone strength.

Readers are empowered with knowledge about potential side effects and the importance of regular monitoring and follow-up with healthcare professionals. Alternative and natural treatment options are also discussed for those seeking holistic approaches.

The book then transitions into a discussion of the broader lifestyle changes necessary for optimal bone health. Practical advice on quitting smoking, reducing alcohol consumption, and maintaining an active lifestyle provides readers with actionable steps they can take to improve bone health.

When it comes to managing fractures, the book provides crucial information on how osteoporosis increases the likelihood of fractures and how to address them. It guides readers through the recovery process, the importance of physical therapy, and ways to prevent future fractures. This section also offers practical advice on how to modify one's living environment to reduce the risk of falls and protect against further injury.

Lastly, the book tackles common myths and misconceptions about osteoporosis. It dispels the idea that osteoporosis is a normal part of aging or that it only affects women, providing reassurance that the condition can be managed effectively with proper care. By addressing concerns about exercise, diet, and the potential reversibility of osteoporosis, the book provides clear answers to frequently asked questions, offering readers the knowledge they need to navigate their condition with confidence.

This comprehensive guide stands as an invaluable resource for anyone concerned about osteoporosis, providing detailed information on prevention, management, and the steps needed to lead a healthy, active life despite the challenges of osteoporosis.

Table of Contents

About This Book 4
Introduction 23
    Definition and Causes of Osteoporosis 23
    Key Risk Factors (Age, Genetics, Lifestyle) 24
    Importance of Early Detection 25
    Impact of Osteoporosis on Quality of Life 26
    Why Bone Density Matters 27
Why Prevention is Crucial 28
    The Significance of Bone Health in Aging 28
    Long-Term Consequences of Untreated Osteoporosis 29
    Prevention as a Lifelong Commitment 29
    Key Preventative Strategies (Diet, Exercise, Medication) 30

Role of Healthcare Professionals in Prevention 31
CHAPTER 1: 33
Bone Health Basics 33
What bones are made of: minerals and cells 33
The bone remodeling process 34
Peak bone mass and its importance 35
Hormones that affect bone health 36
Role of calcium and Vitamin D in bone strength.................................37
Understanding bone density tests.38
Osteoporosis vs. osteopenia: what's the difference?...............................39
How bones change with age..........40
Role of genetics in bone health 40
Impact of gender on bone strength (men vs. women) 41
How lifestyle affects bone health ..42

Common myths about bone health 43

Importance of regular check-ups .. 44

CHAPTER 2: 45

Risk Factors for Osteoporosis 45

Age-Related Bone Loss 45

Family History of Osteoporosis 46

Hormonal Imbalances (Menopause and Andropause) 47

Medications that Can Affect Bone Density 48

Lifestyle Factors: Smoking and Alcohol Use 49

Lack of Physical Activity 49

Poor Diet Lacking in Essential Nutrients 50

Medical Conditions That Impact Bone Health 51

Gender and Bone Density Risks 52

Impact of Low Body Weight 52

- Role of Certain Autoimmune Disorders 53
- How Chronic Illnesses Contribute to Bone Weakness 54
- Importance of Recognizing Risk Factors Early 55

CHAPTER 3: 56

Essential Nutrients for Bone Health . 56
- Importance of Calcium for Bone Strength 56
- Role of Vitamin D in Calcium Absorption 57
- Magnesium and Its Effect on Bone Density 58
- Foods Rich in Bone-Supporting Nutrients 58
- Supplements: When and How to Use Them 59
- Best Dietary Sources of Calcium ... 60
- How Vitamin K Supports Bone Health 61

- Importance of Balanced Protein Intake 61
- Hydration and Its Role in Bone Health 62
- Benefits of Dairy vs. Non-Dairy Sources of Calcium 63
- Impact of Caffeine and Salt on Bone Density 64
- Understanding Fortified Foods for Bone Health 64
- Bone-Boosting Meal Ideas 65

CHAPTER 4: 66

Exercise for Strong Bones.................. 66
- Why Weight-Bearing Exercise Matters.. 66
- Best Types of Exercise for Bone Health.. 67
- How Strength Training Improves Bone Density 67
- Safe Exercises for People with Osteoporosis 68

 Importance of Balance Exercises to Prevent Falls 69

 How Walking Improves Bone Strength 70

 The Role of Flexibility in Bone Health 70

 Setting Realistic Exercise Goals.....71

 Benefits of High-Impact Exercises 72

 How Yoga and Pilates Can Help with Bone Health....................................72

 When to Consult a Physical Therapist 73

 Frequency and Duration of Exercise for Optimal Results.......................74

 Overcoming Exercise Barriers for Beginners 75

CHAPTER 5:..76
Medical Treatments and Medications 76

 Overview of Osteoporosis Medications 76

How Bisphosphonates Work 77
Hormone Therapy and Its Role 78
Selective Estrogen Receptor Modulators (SERMs) 79
Role of Calcium and Vitamin D Supplements 80
Injectable Treatments for Osteoporosis 81
Potential Side Effects of Bone Medications 82
Monitoring Bone Density During Treatment 83
Alternative and Natural Treatments 83
Importance of Regular Follow-Ups with Your Doctor 84
How to Manage Medication Side Effects 85
Medications That Might Weaken Bones 86

- How to Discuss Treatment Options with Your Doctor 87
- CHAPTER 6: 88
- Lifestyle Changes for Bone Health 88
  - Quit Smoking for Better Bone Density 88
  - Limiting Alcohol to Protect Bones 89
  - Benefits of a Balanced Diet Rich in Nutrients 90
  - The Importance of Regular Physical Activity 91
  - Managing Stress for Better Overall Health 92
  - Sleep and Its Impact on Bone Regeneration 93
  - Staying Active in Older Age 93
  - How Weight Loss Affects Bone Health 94
  - Managing Chronic Conditions That Impact Bones 95

- Maintaining a Healthy Body Weight 96
- How to Build Healthy Habits 96
- Staying Motivated in Your Bone Health Journey 97
- How to Avoid Injury and Protect Your Bones 98

CHAPTER 7: 99
Managing Fractures and Bone Injuries 99

- How Osteoporosis Leads to Fractures 99
- Signs and Symptoms of a Bone Fracture..100
- How Fractures Are Diagnosed.....101
- Common Sites for Osteoporosis Fractures (Spine, Hip, Wrist) 102
- Recovery Process After a Fracture 103
- How to Prevent Future Fractures104

    Physical Therapy for Fracture Recovery 105

    Pain Management for Bone Injuries 106

    Importance of Rehabilitation Exercises 107

    How to Modify Your Home to Prevent Falls 108

    Role of Assistive Devices (Canes, Walkers) 109

    When Surgery Is Necessary for Fractures 110

    Long-Term Outlook for Bone Injury Recovery 111

CHAPTER 8: 112

Common Concerns and Myths about Osteoporosis 112

    Is Osteoporosis a Normal Part of Aging? 112

    Does Only Women Get Osteoporosis? 113

Can Diet Alone Prevent Osteoporosis? 114

Is Exercise Too Risky for People with Osteoporosis? 114

Do Fractures Heal Completely in People with Osteoporosis? 115

Is Osteoporosis Only a Concern After Menopause? 116

Can Osteoporosis Be Reversed with Treatment? 117

Are Supplements Enough to Protect Bones? 118

Is Bone Loss Always Noticeable? . 119

Can Osteoporosis Medications Harm Other Parts of the Body? 119

Is Weight Training Safe for Osteoporosis Patients? 120

Does Being Active Mean You Won't Get Osteoporosis? 121

Can Young People Develop Osteoporosis? 122

CHAPTER 9: 123

Frequently Asked Questions (FAQs) 123

What is the best test for diagnosing osteoporosis? 123

At what age should I start getting tested for bone density? 124

How much calcium and Vitamin D do I need daily? 125

Can I build back bone once it's lost? 125

What are the side effects of osteoporosis medications? 126

How often should I get a bone density test? 127

Are men at risk for osteoporosis? 128

What type of doctor treats osteoporosis? 128

Is osteoporosis painful? 129

How do I know if my exercise routine is helping my bones? 130

Can children develop osteoporosis? 131

How long will I need to take osteoporosis medication? 131

Can diet alone manage osteoporosis? 132

Conclusion 133

Introduction

Definition and Causes of Osteoporosis

Osteoporosis is a medical condition where bones become weak and brittle, making them more susceptible to fractures. It occurs when the creation of new bone doesn't keep up with the removal of old bone. As a result, bones lose density and strength, which increases the risk of breaks even from minor stresses. Commonly affecting older adults, especially postmenopausal women, it is often referred to as a "silent disease" because bone loss occurs without obvious symptoms until a fracture happens.

The main causes of osteoporosis include a decrease in bone-building hormones (like estrogen in women and testosterone in men), aging, inadequate intake of calcium and vitamin D, and lack of physical activity. Other causes can be long-term use of corticosteroids, excessive alcohol consumption, and certain chronic medical conditions such as thyroid disorders or gastrointestinal diseases that affect nutrient absorption.

Key Risk Factors (Age, Genetics, Lifestyle)

Age is the biggest risk factor for osteoporosis, as bone density naturally decreases as people get older. After age 30, bone mass starts to decline, and women are particularly vulnerable after menopause due to a significant drop in estrogen levels. Genetics also plays a role; if osteoporosis runs in your family, you're more likely to develop the condition yourself.

Lifestyle factors significantly impact bone health as well. Smoking, excessive alcohol consumption, and a sedentary lifestyle increase the risk of osteoporosis. A poor diet, especially one low in calcium and vitamin D, weakens bones over time. Conversely, regular weight-bearing exercise like walking, running, or resistance training can help strengthen bones and reduce the risk.

Importance of Early Detection

Detecting osteoporosis early is crucial because bone loss can happen without noticeable symptoms. The earlier osteoporosis is identified, the better the chances of slowing or halting bone density loss. Bone density tests, such as dual-energy X-ray absorptiometry (DEXA scans), are the standard way to assess bone health. These tests measure the density of bones, particularly in the spine and hips, where fractures are most common.

Getting a DEXA scan is a simple, non-invasive procedure that can identify low bone density before fractures occur. Doctors typically recommend these tests for women over 65 and men over 70, or earlier if there are significant risk factors such as family history or long-term steroid use. With early detection, a combination of lifestyle changes, supplements, and medications can help manage bone health.

Impact of Osteoporosis on Quality of Life

Osteoporosis can significantly impact a person's quality of life due to the increased risk of fractures, especially in the spine, hips, and wrists. Even minor falls or injuries can lead to broken bones, resulting in chronic pain, disability, and a reduced ability to perform everyday tasks. Fractures can also lead to long recovery periods, loss of independence, and emotional stress.

The psychological effects of osteoporosis should not be overlooked. Fear of falling and the possibility of breaking a bone can cause older adults to avoid physical activity, further weakening bones and muscles. This can create a cycle of inactivity and isolation, leading to a decline in overall health and well-being.

Why Bone Density Matters

Bone density is a critical measure of bone strength and overall bone health. Higher bone density means that bones are stronger and less likely to fracture. Maintaining or improving bone density is essential, especially as people age. Weight-bearing exercises like walking, dancing, or resistance training help stimulate bone formation and slow down the natural process of bone loss.

A healthy diet rich in calcium, vitamin D, and other essential nutrients also plays a key role in maintaining bone density. Calcium is the building block of bone tissue, while vitamin D helps the body absorb calcium effectively. Adequate intake of these nutrients, combined with an active lifestyle, can help preserve bone density and reduce the risk of osteoporosis and fractures.

Why Prevention is Crucial

The Significance of Bone Health in Aging

As we age, our bones naturally lose density, becoming more fragile and susceptible to fractures. This is due to the body's reduced ability to rebuild bone tissue, making bone health a critical focus for older adults. Weak bones can lead to debilitating issues like fractures, limiting mobility and independence, and increasing the risk of complications such as prolonged hospital stays.

Maintaining strong bones is essential for overall well-being. Key lifestyle choices such as regular exercise, a balanced diet rich in calcium and vitamin D, and minimizing alcohol and smoking can go a long way in preserving bone health. Strengthening bones helps ensure better balance, mobility, and quality of life in later years.

Long-Term Consequences of Untreated Osteoporosis

Osteoporosis is a silent disease, often progressing without symptoms until a fracture occurs. Left untreated, it can lead to severe complications like hip fractures, spinal deformities, and chronic pain. These fractures not only impair movement but can also cause long-term disability, reducing independence.

If osteoporosis is not managed, individuals may face frequent fractures from minor falls, increasing hospital visits, and the need for assisted living. This makes early detection and treatment crucial in preventing these life-altering consequences.

Prevention as a Lifelong Commitment

Preventing osteoporosis starts early and continues throughout life. Bone mass peaks in the late twenties, and from then on, it's crucial to maintain healthy habits like regular weight-bearing exercise and a diet high in calcium and vitamin D. These practices help delay or even prevent the onset of osteoporosis.

Commitment to bone health means regular checkups, including bone density tests for those at risk, and staying informed about changes in health as we age. Being proactive ensures that bone health remains a priority throughout life, significantly reducing the risk of fractures later on.

Key Preventative Strategies (Diet, Exercise, Medication)

A diet rich in calcium (dairy products, leafy greens) and vitamin D (sunlight, fortified foods) is vital for maintaining strong bones. Supplements can be beneficial for those who struggle to meet their nutritional needs through diet alone. Weight-bearing exercises like walking, jogging, and resistance training also help strengthen bones by promoting bone formation.

In cases where diet and exercise are not enough, medications like bisphosphonates, hormone replacement therapy, or calcium supplements may be recommended by a healthcare provider. Combining these strategies provides a comprehensive approach to maintaining bone density and preventing osteoporosis.

Role of Healthcare Professionals in Prevention

Healthcare professionals play a key role in osteoporosis prevention by offering regular bone density screenings, especially for older adults or those at high risk. They can provide personalized advice on diet, exercise, and medication to strengthen bones and reduce the risk of fractures.

Doctors may prescribe medications for those diagnosed with osteoporosis or at high risk, monitor progress, and adjust treatment plans. Regular consultations ensure that patients stay informed about the latest preventive measures and make any necessary lifestyle adjustments for optimal bone health.

CHAPTER 1:

Bone Health Basics

What bones are made of: minerals and cells

Bones are composed of two primary elements: minerals and cells. The hard outer layer, known as cortical bone, is made of minerals like calcium and phosphate, giving bones their strength and rigidity. Inside, bones are more flexible and consist of collagen and living bone cells such as osteoblasts (which build new bone) and osteoclasts (which break down old bone). This combination of minerals and cells allows bones to be both strong and slightly flexible to withstand daily stress.

Additionally, the spongy bone inside, known as trabecular bone, supports the marrow, which produces blood cells. Together, these elements maintain bone structure, repair damage, and store essential minerals. Proper care, including a nutrient-rich diet and exercise, helps keep bones healthy and functioning.

The bone remodeling process

Bone remodeling is a continuous cycle where old bone is broken down, and new bone is formed. This process occurs throughout life and is critical for maintaining bone strength. Osteoclasts remove old, weakened bone, creating small cavities. Then, osteoblasts fill these cavities by producing new bone tissue. This balance keeps bones resilient and capable of repairing micro-damage that occurs from daily activities.

In youth, bone formation exceeds bone breakdown, leading to growth. As we age, this balance can shift, leading to bone loss if breakdown outpaces formation. Maintaining a healthy lifestyle, including adequate calcium intake and regular weight-bearing exercise, supports the remodeling process and helps slow bone loss.

Peak bone mass and its importance

Peak bone mass refers to the maximum bone strength and density that a person achieves, typically by their late 20s. This is a crucial time because the higher your peak bone mass, the more bone reserve you have as you age. Achieving high peak bone mass reduces the risk of osteoporosis and fractures later in life.

Building strong bones during childhood and adolescence, through good nutrition (especially calcium and vitamin D) and regular exercise, is key. After peak bone mass is reached, the focus shifts to preserving bone density through lifestyle choices like staying active and ensuring proper nutrient intake.

Hormones that affect bone health

Several hormones play significant roles in regulating bone health. Estrogen is crucial in women, as it helps maintain bone density. After menopause, estrogen levels drop, leading to an increased risk of osteoporosis. Testosterone also supports bone health in men, although its effects are less pronounced than estrogen's role in women. Parathyroid hormone regulates calcium levels in the blood, directly influencing bone remodeling.

Additionally, calcitonin helps reduce bone resorption, while growth hormone and insulin-like growth factors promote bone formation. Managing hormonal changes, particularly after menopause, with lifestyle adjustments or medical treatments can help preserve bone density.

Role of calcium and Vitamin D in bone strength

Calcium is the building block of bones, providing them with the strength and density they need to function. Without enough calcium, bones become weak and brittle. Vitamin D, on the other hand, helps the body absorb calcium from food and supplements. Without sufficient Vitamin D, even with adequate calcium intake, bones cannot effectively maintain their density.

To support bone health, aim for a diet rich in calcium from sources like dairy products, leafy greens, and fortified foods. Regular sunlight exposure or Vitamin D supplements are also essential, especially in older adults, to ensure calcium absorption.

Understanding bone density tests

Bone density tests measure the strength and thickness of bones to assess the risk of fractures and diagnose conditions like osteoporosis. The most common test is the DEXA scan, which uses low levels of X-rays to measure bone mineral density in areas like the spine and hips. Results are compared to the bone density of a healthy young adult, giving a T-score that indicates normal bone density, osteopenia (low bone mass), or osteoporosis.

Bone density tests are simple, non-invasive, and critical for early detection of bone issues, allowing for timely treatment. Regular testing, especially for postmenopausal women and older adults, can help manage bone health and prevent fractures.

Osteoporosis vs. osteopenia: what's the difference?

Osteoporosis and osteopenia both refer to reduced bone density, but they differ in severity. Osteopenia is a condition where bone density is lower than normal, but not low enough to be classified as osteoporosis. It's a warning sign that bones are weakening, but the risk of fractures is not as high as in osteoporosis.

Osteoporosis is a more serious condition where bone density is significantly decreased, making bones fragile and more prone to fractures. Both conditions can be managed with lifestyle changes, medications, and regular monitoring, but osteoporosis requires more aggressive treatment to prevent serious complications.

How bones change with age

As we age, our bones naturally lose density and strength. In early adulthood, bone remodeling is balanced, but starting around age 30, bone breakdown begins to outpace formation. This leads to a gradual loss of bone mass. In women, bone loss accelerates after menopause due to decreased estrogen levels, increasing the risk of osteoporosis.

Bone loss affects both men and women, though it tends to occur later in men. To slow the effects of aging on bones, regular weight-bearing exercise, a calcium-rich diet, and avoiding smoking and excessive alcohol are essential.

Role of genetics in bone health

Genetics play a key role in determining an individual's bone density and risk of developing osteoporosis. If your parents or siblings have a history of osteoporosis or fractures, you may have a higher genetic risk of experiencing similar issues. Your genetic makeup can influence factors such as peak bone mass, bone turnover rates, and how your body uses calcium.

While you can't change your genetic predisposition, understanding your family history allows you to take proactive steps. Regular exercise, a nutrient-rich diet, and medical screenings can help mitigate genetic risks and maintain bone health.

Impact of gender on bone strength (men vs. women)

Women generally have smaller, thinner bones than men, making them more prone to bone density loss as they age. After menopause, the sharp decline in estrogen levels accelerates bone loss, increasing the risk of osteoporosis. This is why women are four times more likely than men to develop the condition.

Men also experience bone loss with age, but it typically occurs more gradually due to slower testosterone decline. While men are less likely to develop osteoporosis, they should still focus on maintaining bone health through diet, exercise, and regular screenings, especially after age 50.

How lifestyle affects bone health

Lifestyle choices have a profound impact on bone health. A sedentary lifestyle can weaken bones, while regular weight-bearing activities like walking, jogging, or strength training can help maintain bone density. Smoking and excessive alcohol consumption increase bone loss, while a balanced diet rich in calcium and Vitamin D promotes strong bones.

Maintaining a healthy weight is also essential. Being underweight can lead to bone loss, while being overweight increases stress on bones, especially in the joints. Adopting healthy habits early can significantly reduce the risk of bone-related issues later in life.

Common myths about bone health

A common myth is that only women need to worry about osteoporosis. While women are at higher risk, men can also develop the condition, especially as they age. Another myth is that if you're young, you don't need to think about your bone health. In reality, building strong bones in your youth sets the foundation for bone health later in life.

Some also believe that taking calcium supplements alone will prevent osteoporosis. While calcium is crucial, it needs to be paired with adequate Vitamin D, exercise, and other nutrients to be effective. Understanding these misconceptions can help people take a more holistic approach to bone care.

Importance of regular check-ups

Regular check-ups are vital for maintaining bone health, especially as you age. Bone density tests, such as DEXA scans, can detect early signs of bone loss, allowing for timely intervention. Blood tests can also monitor levels of calcium, Vitamin D, and other markers of bone health, helping prevent or manage conditions like osteoporosis.

Discussing risk factors, such as family history, lifestyle habits, or hormonal changes, with your doctor is essential for personalized care. Regular medical evaluations ensure that any issues are caught early, making treatment more effective and reducing the risk of fractures.

CHAPTER 2:

Risk Factors for Osteoporosis

Age-Related Bone Loss

As we age, bones naturally lose density, making them more fragile and prone to fractures. This is because the body's ability to produce new bone cells slows down, and bone breakdown occurs more quickly than bone formation. For older adults, regular weight-bearing exercises like walking or lifting light weights can help slow down this bone loss and improve bone strength.

Along with exercise, ensuring a diet rich in calcium and vitamin D is essential. These nutrients help in the absorption and strengthening of bones, supporting the body in replenishing lost bone density. Regular bone density tests are recommended for older adults to monitor changes and take preventive action early.

Family History of Osteoporosis

Osteoporosis can be hereditary, and a family history of the condition increases the risk of developing it. If a parent or sibling has been diagnosed with osteoporosis or has experienced fractures from minor falls, it's important to inform your healthcare provider. This information allows for early screening and preventive measures to reduce bone loss risk.

To mitigate this inherited risk, maintain an active lifestyle with regular strength training exercises and ensure sufficient intake of bone-boosting nutrients like calcium, vitamin D, and magnesium. Early lifestyle changes, combined with medical monitoring, can reduce the likelihood of osteoporosis even with a genetic predisposition.

Hormonal Imbalances (Menopause and Andropause)

Menopause in women and andropause in men both lead to a significant drop in hormones like estrogen and testosterone, which are crucial for maintaining bone density. Women, particularly post-menopausal, are more vulnerable to rapid bone loss due to decreased estrogen levels, which protect bones.

To manage this, hormone replacement therapy (HRT) is sometimes recommended by doctors to maintain hormonal balance and support bone health. Additionally, exercises that strengthen bones and joints, along with a diet rich in bone-supporting nutrients, can help mitigate the effects of hormonal changes on bone density.

Medications that Can Affect Bone Density

Certain medications, such as corticosteroids or anticonvulsants, can weaken bones by interfering with the body's ability to absorb calcium or by increasing bone breakdown. If you're on long-term medications, it's essential to discuss bone health with your doctor and explore alternatives or supplements that can minimize the risk of bone density loss.

Regular bone density scans and a preventive diet high in calcium and vitamin D are vital for individuals on these medications. Weight-bearing exercises, such as yoga or resistance training, also support bone health and counteract the negative effects of these drugs.

Lifestyle Factors: Smoking and Alcohol Use

Smoking and excessive alcohol consumption significantly contribute to bone loss. Smoking reduces the body's ability to absorb calcium, while alcohol impairs bone formation. Both habits speed up the bone-aging process, leading to weaker, brittle bones.

Quitting smoking and limiting alcohol intake can greatly reduce the risk of osteoporosis. Replacing these habits with healthier lifestyle choices, such as regular physical activity and a nutrient-rich diet, helps improve bone health and density over time.

Lack of Physical Activity

Sedentary lifestyles can lead to faster bone loss because bones need regular movement and resistance to stay strong. Without physical activity, bones can weaken, increasing the risk of fractures.

Simple weight-bearing exercises like walking, running, or climbing stairs stimulate bone cells, helping to maintain or increase bone density.

Incorporating strength training, such as using resistance bands or light weights, into your daily routine strengthens muscles and bones, promoting better balance and reducing the likelihood of falls and fractures.

Poor Diet Lacking in Essential Nutrients

A diet lacking in calcium, vitamin D, magnesium, and protein can accelerate bone loss, making bones brittle and prone to fractures. Calcium and vitamin D are particularly important for bone health as they work together to maintain bone density and structure.

To support bone health, include foods rich in calcium like dairy products, leafy greens, and fortified foods in your diet. Supplementing with vitamin D, particularly in regions with low sunlight, ensures better calcium absorption. Also, avoid excessive sodium and caffeine, which can lead to calcium loss from the bones.

Medical Conditions That Impact Bone Health

Certain medical conditions, such as rheumatoid arthritis or thyroid disorders, can negatively affect bone density. These conditions cause inflammation or hormonal imbalances that accelerate bone loss and increase the risk of fractures.

Managing these conditions through medication and lifestyle adjustments is crucial. Regular exercise, along with a diet high in bone-strengthening nutrients, can help minimize bone damage. Monitoring bone density regularly allows for timely interventions, including medications that help preserve bone mass.

Gender and Bone Density Risks

Women are generally more susceptible to osteoporosis than men, particularly after menopause due to reduced estrogen levels. However, men are not immune; low testosterone levels in older men can also lead to bone loss. Men may experience a slower rate of bone density loss but are still at significant risk as they age.

Both men and women should engage in strength-training exercises and consume sufficient calcium and vitamin D to maintain bone density. Regular checkups and bone scans are important for early detection and preventive treatment.

Impact of Low Body Weight

Being underweight, especially for older adults, increases the risk of osteoporosis. Lower body weight often correlates with lower bone density, which leaves bones more fragile and prone to fractures. Additionally, people with lower body weight often have lower muscle mass, reducing the support and protection for their bones.

To combat this, a balanced diet that supports both muscle and bone health is crucial. Gaining weight through healthy means, such as consuming nutrient-dense foods and incorporating strength exercises, can improve both bone and overall physical health.

Role of Certain Autoimmune Disorders

Autoimmune disorders such as lupus or celiac disease can lead to bone loss. These conditions can cause chronic inflammation or impair the body's ability to absorb essential nutrients like calcium and vitamin D, which are vital for bone health.

Managing autoimmune conditions with the help of a healthcare provider and adopting an anti-inflammatory diet rich in bone-supporting nutrients can help reduce bone damage. Regular bone density testing is recommended for early detection and treatment of osteoporosis in people with autoimmune diseases.

How Chronic Illnesses Contribute to Bone Weakness

Chronic illnesses, such as diabetes and kidney disease, can lead to poor bone health by interfering with the body's ability to maintain proper calcium and phosphorus levels. These imbalances weaken bones over time, increasing the risk of fractures.

Proper management of chronic illnesses through medication, diet, and exercise is essential to maintaining bone health. Ensuring the intake of adequate calcium and vitamin D can support bone density, while regular medical checkups help monitor and mitigate bone loss caused by chronic conditions.

Importance of Recognizing Risk Factors Early

Identifying risk factors for osteoporosis early on is critical for preventing severe bone loss and fractures. Factors such as family history, hormonal changes, or lifestyle habits (like smoking) can significantly impact bone health if not addressed.

Early screening, adopting healthy lifestyle habits like regular exercise, and ensuring a nutrient-rich diet can help slow or prevent the onset of osteoporosis. Proactive measures, such as regular bone density tests and early treatment, are essential to maintaining strong, healthy bones.

CHAPTER 3:

Essential Nutrients for Bone Health

Importance of Calcium for Bone Strength

Calcium is the primary mineral responsible for building and maintaining strong bones. It helps form the structure of bones and teeth, making them resilient and less likely to fracture. As we age, bone density naturally decreases, so ensuring sufficient calcium intake is crucial to prevent conditions like osteoporosis.

To maintain optimal bone strength, adults should consume around 1,000 to 1,200 mg of calcium daily. This can be achieved by incorporating calcium-rich foods such as dairy, leafy greens, and fortified plant-based milk into the diet. Regular calcium intake, combined with physical activity, supports lifelong bone health.

Role of Vitamin D in Calcium Absorption

Vitamin D plays a crucial role in calcium absorption, ensuring that the calcium consumed through food is properly utilized by the body. Without sufficient Vitamin D, the body struggles to absorb calcium, leading to weakened bones and a higher risk of fractures.

Vitamin D can be obtained from sunlight, fortified foods, and supplements. Spending 10-30 minutes in the sun daily and consuming foods like fatty fish, eggs, and fortified dairy products helps maintain adequate Vitamin D levels, supporting overall bone health.

Magnesium and Its Effect on Bone Density

Magnesium is essential for activating Vitamin D, which in turn helps the body absorb calcium. It plays a critical role in converting Vitamin D into its active form, thereby promoting bone density and strength. A deficiency in magnesium can lead to weaker bones over time.

Magnesium is abundant in foods like leafy greens, nuts, seeds, and whole grains. Incorporating these foods into daily meals can improve bone density, prevent bone deterioration, and ensure that calcium is effectively absorbed and utilized.

Foods Rich in Bone-Supporting Nutrients

To support bone health, a diet rich in nutrients such as calcium, magnesium, Vitamin D, and Vitamin K is essential. These nutrients work together to maintain strong, healthy bones and reduce the risk of bone-related conditions like osteoporosis.

Foods such as leafy greens, nuts, seeds, fatty fish, and dairy products are packed with bone-supporting nutrients. Incorporating a variety of these foods into your daily meals ensures a steady supply of the vitamins and minerals your bones need to stay healthy.

Supplements: When and How to Use Them

Supplements can be beneficial when dietary intake of key nutrients like calcium, Vitamin D, or magnesium is insufficient. It is important to consult a healthcare provider to determine if supplements are necessary and to avoid excessive consumption, which can cause adverse effects.

Calcium and Vitamin D supplements are commonly recommended for older adults or those at risk of osteoporosis. These should be taken as directed, usually with meals, to enhance absorption and ensure the nutrients support bone health effectively.

Best Dietary Sources of Calcium

Calcium-rich foods are essential for maintaining bone strength and preventing bone loss. Dairy products such as milk, cheese, and yogurt are excellent sources of calcium, providing easily absorbable forms of the mineral.

For those who are lactose intolerant or prefer non-dairy options, foods like almonds, tofu, fortified plant-based milk, and leafy greens such as kale and spinach are also great sources of calcium. Including these foods in daily meals helps meet calcium needs for optimal bone health.

How Vitamin K Supports Bone Health

Vitamin K is essential for bone health as it plays a role in binding calcium to the bone matrix, thereby improving bone density. Without adequate Vitamin K, bones can become more brittle and prone to fractures.

Foods rich in Vitamin K include leafy greens like spinach, kale, and broccoli. Consuming these vegetables regularly can enhance bone strength and reduce the risk of osteoporosis, especially in older adults.

Importance of Balanced Protein Intake

Protein is a key component of bone tissue, and consuming enough of it is crucial for maintaining bone strength and preventing bone loss. However, excessive protein can lead to calcium loss through urine, so balance is key.

Good sources of protein include lean meats, fish, eggs, dairy, legumes, and nuts. Aim for a balanced intake to support bone structure while also ensuring that calcium levels remain stable, promoting overall bone health.

Hydration and Its Role in Bone Health

Staying hydrated is vital for bone health as water helps transport nutrients like calcium to the bones. Dehydration can impair the body's ability to absorb and utilize essential minerals, weakening bones over time.

Drinking at least 8 glasses of water a day helps maintain hydration and supports the body's ability to nourish bones with the necessary nutrients.

Herbal teas, broths, and water-rich fruits and vegetables can also contribute to proper hydration.

Benefits of Dairy vs. Non-Dairy Sources of Calcium

Dairy products like milk, cheese, and yogurt are traditional sources of calcium, providing a bioavailable form that is easily absorbed by the body. These foods are often fortified with Vitamin D, further enhancing calcium absorption.

Non-dairy sources such as fortified plant-based milk, tofu, almonds, and leafy greens also provide ample calcium. For those who avoid dairy, incorporating these foods ensures adequate calcium intake while supporting bone health just as effectively.

Impact of Caffeine and Salt on Bone Density

Excessive caffeine and salt intake can interfere with calcium absorption and contribute to bone density loss. Caffeine increases calcium excretion through urine, while high salt levels can lead to reduced calcium retention in the body.

To protect bone health, it's recommended to limit caffeine to moderate levels (about 1-2 cups of coffee per day) and reduce salt intake by avoiding processed foods and excessive seasoning. Opt for herbs and spices to enhance flavor without compromising calcium levels.

Understanding Fortified Foods for Bone Health

Fortified foods, such as plant-based milk, orange juice, and cereals, are enhanced with key nutrients like calcium, Vitamin D, and magnesium. These foods offer a convenient way to boost nutrient intake, especially for those who may not get enough from their regular diet.

Including fortified foods in your diet can help bridge the nutritional gaps that may arise from dietary restrictions or preferences, ensuring that your bones receive the support they need for long-term health.

Bone-Boosting Meal Ideas

A bone-boosting meal might include a spinach and tofu stir-fry, providing calcium, magnesium, and Vitamin K, paired with a fortified plant-based milk smoothie for an extra dose of Vitamin D and calcium.

For breakfast, consider oatmeal topped with almonds and fortified orange juice. These meals are not only rich in bone-supporting nutrients but are also easy to prepare, helping maintain strong bones in a practical, tasty way.

CHAPTER 4:

Exercise for Strong Bones

Why Weight-Bearing Exercise Matters

Weight-bearing exercises are crucial for improving bone density because they force your bones to work against gravity, stimulating bone cells to strengthen and grow. These exercises include activities like walking, jogging, and climbing stairs, where your body supports its own weight. Over time, they help slow bone loss, maintain current bone mass, and reduce the risk of fractures.

For beginners, start with simple activities like brisk walking or light hiking. Gradually increase the intensity or duration as you build stamina. Weight-bearing exercises should become part of your routine to ensure your bones remain strong and healthy, especially as you age.

Best Types of Exercise for Bone Health

The best exercises for bone health combine weight-bearing and strength training activities. Weight-bearing exercises include walking, dancing, and tennis, while strength training uses resistance to build muscles and bones through exercises like squats, lunges, and lifting weights.

A practical approach is to combine these two types of exercises weekly. For instance, aim for 30 minutes of walking five days a week and two sessions of strength training. This combination strengthens both your bones and muscles, reducing the risk of osteoporosis.

How Strength Training Improves Bone Density

Strength training improves bone density by creating controlled stress on your bones, which encourages them to grow stronger. Using resistance bands, free weights, or machines, you target a specific muscle group, which in turn stimulates bone growth in those areas.

To start, perform exercises like squats, deadlifts, or push-ups using your body weight or light dumbbells. As you progress, gradually increase the weight or resistance. This helps build muscle and bone density, reducing the risk of osteoporosis-related fractures.

Safe Exercises for People with Osteoporosis

For individuals with osteoporosis, it's essential to focus on safe, low-impact exercises that improve strength without putting undue stress on fragile bones. Seated leg lifts, standing leg curls, and wall push-ups are effective and safe options.

Start with exercises that don't involve bending forward or twisting the spine, as these movements can increase fracture risk. Focus on slow, controlled movements that build strength, improve balance, and reduce the chance of falls or injuries.

Importance of Balance Exercises to Prevent Falls

Balance exercises are critical for preventing falls, especially for those with osteoporosis, where even a minor fall can result in fractures. Simple exercises like standing on one foot or practicing heel-to-toe walking can improve your stability.

Include balance exercises in your daily routine by starting with 10 minutes a day. Over time, improve your balance by practicing more challenging moves, like standing on one leg while closing your eyes, which will enhance coordination and prevent falls.

How Walking Improves Bone Strength

Walking is an accessible and effective weight-bearing exercise that strengthens bones, especially in the hips and lower body. It encourages the bone to remodel and build density without putting excessive strain on the joints, making it ideal for all fitness levels.

A daily 30-minute brisk walk can significantly contribute to maintaining and improving bone health. Make walking a habit by incorporating it into daily activities, such as walking to the store or taking the stairs, to ensure your bones stay healthy.

The Role of Flexibility in Bone Health

Flexibility exercises improve joint mobility, reducing stiffness and enhancing your ability to perform everyday activities. Stretching regularly helps maintain the elasticity of muscles and tendons around your bones, lowering the risk of injury.

To improve flexibility, incorporate gentle stretches after every workout, focusing on areas like the hips, shoulders, and spine. Yoga poses, such as the cat-cow stretch or child's pose, can help maintain mobility and support bone health.

Setting Realistic Exercise Goals

Setting realistic exercise goals ensures that you stay motivated and progress at a pace that suits your body. Start by defining small, achievable goals, such as walking for 15 minutes daily, then gradually increase the duration and intensity over time.

Break down your long-term fitness goals into weekly or monthly targets. This approach helps you track progress, stay committed, and prevent burnout, ensuring a sustainable routine for improving bone health.

Benefits of High-Impact Exercises

High-impact exercises, like running, jumping, or dancing, place additional stress on bones, stimulating them to become denser and stronger. These activities are particularly beneficial for people with good bone health and those looking to prevent osteoporosis.

For beginners, start with moderate-impact activities like brisk walking or stair climbing. Once you've built stamina, you can gradually incorporate short bursts of jumping or running to further enhance bone density.

How Yoga and Pilates Can Help with Bone Health

Yoga and Pilates improve both flexibility and strength, promoting bone health by engaging muscles that support and stabilize bones. These practices involve slow, controlled movements that enhance posture, balance, and alignment, reducing the risk of falls.

Begin with gentle yoga poses like Warrior I or II, or basic Pilates moves such as leg lifts and core strengthening. These exercises are safe for most people, including those with osteoporosis, and help improve overall bone health and balance.

When to Consult a Physical Therapist

If you have osteoporosis or are at high risk of fractures, consulting a physical therapist can be highly beneficial. A therapist will assess your current physical condition and design a personalized exercise plan that strengthens bones and improves mobility without risking injury.

Seek professional guidance, especially if you're new to exercise or have pre-existing conditions. A therapist can teach you proper techniques, recommend safe exercises, and monitor your progress to ensure you're building bone strength safely.

Frequency and Duration of Exercise for Optimal Results

For optimal bone health, aim for 150 minutes of moderate-weight-bearing exercise weekly, spread over five days. Combine this with strength training exercises twice a week to improve bone density and muscle strength.

Break down your exercise routine into manageable chunks, such as 30-minute daily sessions. Consistency is key, so it's essential to find a routine that fits your lifestyle, ensuring regular activity to maintain and strengthen your bones over time.

Overcoming Exercise Barriers for Beginners

Starting an exercise routine can be daunting, especially for beginners. To overcome barriers, begin with low-impact exercises, such as walking or stretching, and gradually increase the intensity as your fitness improves. Set short-term, achievable goals to maintain motivation.

If time is an issue, incorporate small bursts of activity throughout the day, such as taking the stairs or walking during breaks. The key is consistency; even small steps toward regular exercise can significantly improve your bone health over time.

CHAPTER 5:

Medical Treatments and Medications

Overview of Osteoporosis Medications

Osteoporosis medications primarily focus on slowing down bone loss or promoting bone growth. The most commonly prescribed drugs include bisphosphonates, SERMs, hormone therapy, and inject able treatments. Each of these medications works differently to protect bone density and reduce the risk of fractures. It's important for patients to understand the benefits of each medication and how they work to make informed decisions with their healthcare provider.

Patients should always follow medical advice when taking these medications, which may involve taking them daily, weekly, or even yearly. It's essential to maintain a consistent routine, as missed doses can reduce effectiveness. Understanding the different options available allows for personalized treatment that best suits the patient's needs.

How Bisphosphonates Work

Bisphosphonates are among the most common treatments for osteoporosis. They work by slowing the rate at which bones break down, which helps maintain or increase bone density. These medications bind to the bone surface, preventing bone-resorbing cells (osteoclasts) from breaking down the bone tissue, which can lead to stronger, healthier bones over time.

Typically taken orally or through intravenous infusion, bisphosphonates should be consumed on an empty stomach with water and require remaining upright for at least 30 minutes afterward to prevent esophageal irritation. Long-term use requires regular monitoring to ensure they are still effective and to avoid rare side effects like jaw problems.

Hormone Therapy and Its Role

Hormone therapy is often used in postmenopausal women to manage osteoporosis. Estrogen, which decreases after menopause, plays a vital role in maintaining bone density. Hormone replacement therapy (HRT) works by supplementing estrogen levels, helping slow bone loss and reducing the risk of fractures.

However, hormone therapy comes with potential risks, including an increased chance of breast cancer, stroke, or blood clots. This treatment is often reserved for those with severe osteoporosis or those who cannot tolerate other medications. It's crucial to discuss the benefits and risks of hormone therapy with a healthcare provider before starting treatment.

Selective Estrogen Receptor Modulators (SERMs)

SERMs, like raloxifene, mimic the effects of estrogen on bones without some of the risks associated with hormone therapy. They help reduce bone loss and may even improve bone density in some women, especially those who are postmenopausal.

Taken in pill form, SERMs are generally well tolerated, but they can increase the risk of blood clots. Patients using SERMs should monitor for signs of clotting, like swelling or pain in the legs, and maintain an active lifestyle to promote circulation. SERMs offer an alternative for women who need the benefits of estrogen without the risks associated with hormone therapy.

Role of Calcium and Vitamin D Supplements

Calcium and Vitamin D are crucial nutrients for bone health. Calcium provides the building blocks for strong bones, while Vitamin D helps the body absorb calcium effectively. Most people should aim for a daily intake of 1,000 to 1,200 mg of calcium and 600 to 800 IU of Vitamin D.

These supplements can be taken in tablet form or absorbed through foods like dairy products, leafy greens, and fortified foods. For optimal absorption, take calcium in smaller doses (500 mg or less) throughout the day, preferably with meals. Consistent use of these supplements can help maintain bone density, especially when paired with osteoporosis medications.

Injectable Treatments for Osteoporosis

Injectable treatments like denosumab or teriparatide offer alternatives for people who cannot tolerate oral medications. Denosumab works by preventing bone breakdown, while teriparatide stimulates new bone growth. Both are typically administered via injection, either every six months (denosumab) or daily (teriparatide).

These treatments are usually prescribed for severe osteoporosis cases or for individuals who haven't responded well to other treatments. It's important to follow a strict injection schedule, as missing doses can quickly reduce the medication's effectiveness. Always consult with your doctor about the proper use and monitoring needed for injectable osteoporosis treatments.

Potential Side Effects of Bone Medications

While osteoporosis medications can be effective, they may cause side effects, which vary depending on the drug. Common side effects include gastrointestinal issues like nausea or heartburn (especially with bisphosphonates), headaches, muscle pain, or, in rare cases, more severe conditions like atypical fractures or jaw osteonecrosis.

It's important for patients to report any unusual symptoms to their doctor immediately. Side effects can often be managed by adjusting the dosage, switching medications, or adding supportive treatments. Knowing what to expect allows patients to balance treatment benefits with any potential discomfort.

Monitoring Bone Density During Treatment

Bone density should be monitored regularly to assess how well osteoporosis treatment is working. A DEXA scan (dual-energy X-ray absorptiometry) is the most common way to measure bone density. These scans are typically done every one to two years, depending on the treatment plan.

Regular monitoring helps adjust medications if needed. If bone density is decreasing despite treatment, your doctor may recommend a different medication or additional supplements. Staying on top of your bone health through regular scans ensures that your treatment remains effective over time.

Alternative and Natural Treatments

Alternative treatments for osteoporosis include lifestyle changes like improving diet, increasing physical activity, and incorporating supplements such as magnesium, Vitamin K, and omega-3 fatty acids. Weight-bearing exercises like walking, resistance training, and yoga can also strengthen bones naturally.

Some people turn to herbal remedies or acupuncture, though these should always be discussed with a healthcare provider. While alternative treatments can support overall health, they should complement, not replace, traditional medical treatments, especially for individuals with high fracture risk.

Importance of Regular Follow-Ups with Your Doctor

Regular follow-ups are crucial for those managing osteoporosis. These check-ins allow doctors to assess how well medications are working, review bone density scans, and make any necessary adjustments to the treatment plan. Follow-up appointments usually occur every six months to a year.

In addition to monitoring bone health, follow-ups provide an opportunity to discuss any new symptoms, side effects, or lifestyle changes that could affect your treatment. Consistent communication with your doctor ensures that osteoporosis management stays on track and effective.

How to Manage Medication Side Effects

Managing medication side effects involves understanding the common reactions associated with osteoporosis drugs and taking steps to mitigate them. For instance, taking bisphosphonates with plenty of water and staying upright can reduce gastrointestinal discomfort. Additionally, patients may switch to a different medication if side effects become intolerable.

In some cases, doctors may recommend lifestyle changes, such as dietary adjustments or physical activity, to counteract side effects like muscle or joint pain. Open communication with healthcare providers is key to finding the right balance between effective treatment and manageable side effects.

Medications That Might Weaken Bones

Certain medications, such as corticosteroids, can weaken bones and increase the risk of osteoporosis. Long-term use of drugs like prednisone can interfere with bone-building cells, leading to decreased bone density over time.

If you're taking medications that could weaken your bones, it's important to discuss this with your doctor. They may prescribe bone-strengthening treatments or suggest lifestyle changes to counteract these effects, such as increasing calcium and

Vitamin D intake or engaging in regular weight-bearing exercises.

How to Discuss Treatment Options with Your Doctor

When discussing treatment options with your doctor, it's essential to be informed and ask about the benefits and risks of each medication. Patients should inquire about how each option works, its side effects, and any potential long-term consequences. Be open about any concerns, medical history, or preferences for treatment.

Having a clear understanding of your goals, such as preventing fractures or maintaining mobility, will help guide the conversation. Collaborate with your doctor to create a personalized plan that aligns with your health needs, lifestyle, and risk factors.

CHAPTER 6:

Lifestyle Changes for Bone Health

Quit Smoking for Better Bone Density

Quitting smoking is essential for maintaining strong bones. Smoking reduces calcium absorption, weakens bones, and increases the risk of osteoporosis. To quit, start by seeking support from healthcare providers, nicotine replacement therapies, or counseling services. Gradually reduce smoking, set a quit date, and stick to it, as bone density begins to improve when smoking is stopped.

Incorporating bone-strengthening habits like consuming calcium-rich foods and vitamin D supplements can further enhance bone density after quitting. Engage in regular weight-bearing exercises like walking or resistance training to boost bone strength, helping to reverse some of the damage caused by smoking.

Limiting Alcohol to Protect Bones

Alcohol can interfere with the body's ability to absorb calcium, leading to weaker bones over time. To protect bone health, limit alcohol intake to no more than one drink per day for women and two for men. Gradually reduce consumption by replacing alcoholic drinks with non-alcoholic alternatives and keeping track of daily intake.

Pair this reduction with lifestyle changes like increasing intake of calcium-rich foods and engaging in regular exercise. This combination supports bone health while limiting alcohol's negative impact, making it easier to prevent bone-related issues such as fractures and osteoporosis.

Benefits of a Balanced Diet Rich in Nutrients

A balanced diet plays a crucial role in maintaining bone health. Focus on consuming calcium-rich foods like dairy, leafy greens, and fortified products. Ensure you also get enough vitamin D from sunlight or supplements to aid calcium absorption. Other nutrients like magnesium and potassium found in nuts, seeds, and fruits are also important for bone strength.

Pairing this nutrient-rich diet with regular physical activity like resistance exercises maximizes bone health benefits. Simple changes, like eating more whole foods and reducing processed food intake, can make a significant difference in preventing osteoporosis and bone fractures.

The Importance of Regular Physical Activity

Regular physical activity, especially weight-bearing and strength-training exercises, is essential for building and maintaining strong bones. Activities like walking, jogging, or lifting weights put stress on the bones, prompting them to rebuild and strengthen. Aim for at least 30 minutes of such activities five times a week.

Consistency is key, and incorporating fun exercises like dancing or yoga can help keep the routine engaging. In addition to building bone mass, exercise improves balance and coordination, reducing the risk of falls and fractures, especially as you age.

Managing Stress for Better Overall Health

Chronic stress can negatively affect bone health by increasing cortisol levels, which weakens bones over time. Managing stress through relaxation techniques such as meditation, deep breathing, or mindfulness can help reduce cortisol production and protect your bones.

Incorporating stress-relieving activities like yoga or leisurely walks into your routine helps lower anxiety and benefits bone health. Combining stress management with other healthy habits, like a balanced diet and regular exercise, creates a holistic approach to maintaining bone strength and overall well-being.

Sleep and Its Impact on Bone Regeneration

Sleep is essential for bone regeneration, as the body repairs and rebuilds bones during deep sleep. To improve bone health, aim for 7-9 hours of quality sleep per night. Establishing a regular sleep schedule and creating a relaxing bedtime routine can help ensure restful sleep.

Ensure your diet includes nutrients like calcium and magnesium, which promote better sleep quality and bone repair. By prioritizing sleep, you can support the natural process of bone regeneration, reducing the risk of osteoporosis and fractures.

Staying Active in Older Age

Staying active as you age is crucial for maintaining bone density and mobility. Engage in low-impact exercises like swimming, walking, or tai chi to stay fit without putting excessive strain on your joints.

These activities help maintain bone strength, improve balance, and reduce the risk of falls.

Incorporate strength training at least twice a week to support muscle and bone health. Keeping a regular exercise routine in older age is key to preventing bone loss, preserving mobility, and promoting overall physical and mental well-being.

How Weight Loss Affects Bone Health

Rapid or excessive weight loss can weaken bones, as the body may lose bone mass along with fat and muscle. If you are trying to lose weight, do so gradually by combining a nutrient-rich diet with strength-building exercises to preserve bone density.

Focus on consuming adequate calcium and vitamin D to support bone health during weight loss. Avoid fad diets that restrict essential nutrients and prioritize a balanced, sustainable eating plan to protect both your bones and your overall health.

Managing Chronic Conditions That Impact Bones

Chronic conditions like diabetes, rheumatoid arthritis, or thyroid disorders can negatively affect bone health. Proper management of these conditions through medication, diet, and exercise is essential to minimizing their impact on bone density.

Work with your healthcare provider to monitor bone health if you have a chronic condition. Include bone-strengthening activities like weight-bearing exercises and ensure you are getting enough calcium and vitamin D to help offset the effects of the chronic condition on your bones.

Maintaining a Healthy Body Weight

Maintaining a healthy body weight is important for bone health. Being underweight increases the risk of bone fractures, while being overweight puts extra stress on your bones. Aim to achieve and maintain a balanced weight through a combination of healthy eating and regular exercise.

Incorporate weight-bearing exercises like walking or light resistance training to strengthen bones. A balanced diet rich in calcium, vitamin D, and protein can further support healthy bones and ensure you maintain a weight that is beneficial for your overall bone health.

How to Build Healthy Habits

Building healthy habits for bone health starts with small, consistent changes. Begin by setting specific goals, such as increasing daily calcium intake or incorporating short, weight-bearing exercise sessions into your routine. Track your progress to stay motivated.

Gradually increase the complexity of these habits as they become part of your lifestyle. Consistency is key, and over time, these small changes can lead to significant improvements in bone health and a reduced risk of fractures or osteoporosis.

Staying Motivated in Your Bone Health Journey

Staying motivated in maintaining bone health can be challenging, but setting achievable goals and celebrating small successes can help. Use reminders and habit-tracking apps to keep yourself accountable and track your progress. Find an exercise routine or physical activities you enjoy, as this increases the likelihood of consistency.

Involve friends or family members in your bone health journey to build support and accountability.

Maintaining motivation is easier when you have a strong network and realistic goals to strive for, making the process of improving bone health more enjoyable and sustainable.

How to Avoid Injury and Protect Your Bones

To avoid injury and protect your bones, focus on activities that improve balance and strength. Incorporate exercises like yoga, tai chi, or resistance training to enhance stability and reduce the risk of falls. Always use proper form during exercise to prevent unnecessary strain on your bones.

Wear protective gear when engaging in higher-risk activities like cycling or contact sports, and ensure your home environment is safe by removing tripping hazards. Regularly engaging in bone-strengthening exercises and taking precautions in daily activities can significantly reduce your risk of injury.

CHAPTER 7:

Managing Fractures and Bone Injuries

How Osteoporosis Leads to Fractures

Osteoporosis is a condition that weakens bones, making them fragile and more susceptible to fractures. As bones lose density, even minor falls or bumps can result in serious injuries, particularly in older adults. The loss of bone tissue occurs silently over time, often without noticeable symptoms until a fracture occurs, which is why awareness and proactive management are crucial.

When the structural integrity of bones is compromised, they can break under stress. This leads to a higher likelihood of fractures occurring, particularly in areas where the bone density is the lowest, such as the spine, hips, and wrists. It is essential to recognize the risk factors, such as aging, hormonal changes, and certain medications, which can exacerbate the likelihood of osteoporosis and, consequently, fractures.

Signs and Symptoms of a Bone Fracture

Identifying the signs of a bone fracture is essential for prompt treatment. Common symptoms include sudden pain at the injury site, swelling, bruising, and difficulty using the affected limb or joint. In some cases, you might notice a deformity or a visible bump where the fracture has occurred. If you experience these symptoms following a fall or injury, it's important to seek medical attention immediately.

Fractures can also present with more subtle signs, such as tenderness when pressure is applied or difficulty bearing weight on the affected area. If you suspect a fracture but it's not visibly apparent, getting an X-ray or other imaging done is crucial to confirm the injury and determine the appropriate treatment plan.

How Fractures Are Diagnosed

Fractures are typically diagnosed through a combination of physical examination and imaging tests. During a physical examination, a healthcare provider will assess the injury, checking for swelling, bruising, and tenderness. They may ask about how the injury occurred and the level of pain experienced to help determine the extent of the damage.

Imaging tests, such as X-rays, are the most common method for diagnosing fractures, as they provide a clear picture of the bone structure. In some cases, advanced imaging techniques like CT scans or MRIs may be necessary to evaluate complex fractures or assess soft tissue damage. Early diagnosis is vital for ensuring effective treatment and promoting healing.

Common Sites for Osteoporosis Fractures (Spine, Hip, Wrist)

Osteoporosis-related fractures most commonly occur in the spine, hips, and wrists due to the vulnerability of these areas. Spinal fractures can lead to significant pain, height loss, and curvature of the spine. It's essential to recognize that vertebral fractures might occur without any noticeable trauma and can manifest as back pain or a change in posture.

Hip fractures are particularly concerning as they often require surgical intervention and can lead to decreased mobility and independence. Wrist fractures, typically occurring from a fall on an outstretched hand, can also result in long-term complications if not treated promptly. Understanding these common fracture sites helps in monitoring and preventing serious injuries in individuals with osteoporosis.

Recovery Process After a Fracture

The recovery process after a fracture involves several stages, beginning with immobilization. Depending on the fracture's severity, you may need a cast or splint to keep the bone in place while it heals. Typically, the healing process can take several weeks to months, during which time it's crucial to follow your healthcare provider's advice regarding activity restrictions.

Physical rehabilitation plays a vital role in recovery. Once your doctor confirms the bone has healed adequately, you can gradually begin rehabilitation exercises. These exercises aim to restore strength and flexibility, helping you regain full function in the affected area and reducing the risk of future fractures.

How to Prevent Future Fractures

Preventing future fractures involves a combination of lifestyle changes and medical interventions. Ensure you maintain a balanced diet rich in calcium and vitamin D, which are vital for bone health. Regular weight-bearing exercises, such as walking, dancing, or resistance training, can help strengthen bones and improve balance, reducing the risk of falls.

Additionally, reviewing medications with your healthcare provider is important, as some can increase fracture risk. If you have been diagnosed with osteoporosis, ask about treatments that can improve bone density and discuss any lifestyle modifications that may enhance your overall bone health.

Physical Therapy for Fracture Recovery

Physical therapy is integral to the recovery process after a fracture, helping to restore mobility and strength. After your doctor assesses that the bone has healed, a physical therapist will create a customized exercise plan tailored to your needs. This may include range-of-motion exercises to improve flexibility and strength training to rebuild muscle around the fracture site.

Attending regular physical therapy sessions can also help you learn safe ways to perform daily activities and prevent future injuries. Your therapist will provide guidance on posture, body mechanics, and exercises that improve balance, significantly contributing to your recovery and overall well-being.

Pain Management for Bone Injuries

Effective pain management is essential during recovery from a bone injury. Over-the-counter pain relievers like acetaminophen or ibuprofen can help alleviate discomfort. If the pain is severe, your doctor may prescribe stronger medications or recommend a combination of therapies, including ice therapy or heat application, to reduce swelling and enhance comfort.

In addition to medication, incorporating relaxation techniques such as deep breathing or gentle stretching can help manage pain levels. Always consult your healthcare provider before starting any new pain management strategy to ensure it aligns with your recovery plan.

Importance of Rehabilitation Exercises

Rehabilitation exercises are crucial for recovering from a fracture and restoring normal function. These exercises help regain strength, flexibility, and range of motion in the injured area. Starting with gentle movements, such as ankle pumps or finger curls, you can progressively increase the intensity as advised by your healthcare provider or physical therapist.

Consistently engaging in rehabilitation exercises can also improve your overall physical health and prevent future injuries. They enhance blood circulation to the area, promote healing, and can reduce stiffness, enabling a smoother transition back to your daily activities.

How to Modify Your Home to Prevent Falls

Modifying your home is vital in preventing falls, especially for individuals with osteoporosis. Start by decluttering spaces and ensuring that pathways are clear. Remove any loose rugs or mats and secure cords or wires that could pose tripping hazards. Installing grab bars in bathrooms and handrails on staircases can also provide added support.

Proper lighting is essential as well; ensure that all areas of your home are well-lit, especially stairs and hallways. Consider using non-slip mats in the bathroom and kitchen to enhance safety. Making these changes can significantly reduce the risk of falls and fractures in your home.

Role of Assistive Devices (Canes, Walkers)

Assistive devices like canes and walkers can greatly enhance stability and mobility for individuals at risk of falls. If you experience difficulty with balance or walking, consult your healthcare provider to determine the most suitable device for your needs. Proper fitting is essential; a cane should reach your wrist when standing upright, while walkers should allow for a comfortable grip.

Using these devices correctly can prevent falls and promote independence in daily activities. Practice using your assistive device in safe environments until you feel comfortable. Remember, these tools are meant to enhance your safety and should be utilized consistently when needed.

When Surgery Is Necessary for Fractures

In some cases, surgery may be necessary to treat fractures, especially when the bone has broken into multiple pieces or is misaligned. Surgical options can include internal fixation (using plates or screws) or external fixation (using rods outside the body). Your healthcare provider will assess the type and location of the fracture to determine the best approach.

Post-surgery, follow your doctor's rehabilitation plan closely to facilitate recovery. This may involve a combination of immobilization and physical therapy to restore function and strength. Being proactive in your recovery will help ensure the best possible outcome after surgical intervention.

Long-Term Outlook for Bone Injury Recovery

The long-term outlook for bone injury recovery can vary based on factors such as age, overall health, and the specific fracture type. Most individuals can expect significant improvement within months, provided they adhere to rehabilitation and care plans. Regular follow-ups with your healthcare provider can help monitor healing and make necessary adjustments to your treatment.

Maintaining a healthy lifestyle, including balanced nutrition and regular exercise, can also positively impact long-term bone health. Staying informed about osteoporosis and implementing preventive measures can minimize future risks, enabling you to lead a more active and fulfilling life.

CHAPTER 8:

Common Concerns and Myths about Osteoporosis

Is Osteoporosis a Normal Part of Aging?

Osteoporosis is not considered an inevitable part of aging, although it is more common in older adults due to the natural decrease in bone density over time. While aging does contribute to the risk of developing osteoporosis, factors such as genetics, lifestyle, and nutrition also play significant roles. Understanding that osteoporosis can be influenced by these modifiable factors is crucial for prevention and management.

To combat age-related bone density loss, individuals can adopt proactive measures such as engaging in weight-bearing exercises and consuming a calcium- and vitamin D-rich diet. By making these lifestyle adjustments early on, older adults can help maintain bone strength and reduce the risk of osteoporosis.

Does Only Women Get Osteoporosis?

While osteoporosis is more prevalent in women, particularly postmenopausal women due to hormonal changes, men can also develop the condition. Approximately one in four men over the age of 50 will experience an osteoporotic fracture. It's essential to recognize that osteoporosis does not discriminate by gender, and awareness should be raised for both men and women.

Men should prioritize bone health by incorporating strength training, maintaining a balanced diet, and getting regular check-ups. Understanding that osteoporosis is a shared concern will encourage both genders to take preventive actions and seek appropriate medical advice.

Can Diet Alone Prevent Osteoporosis?

Diet plays a vital role in bone health, but it cannot single-handedly prevent osteoporosis. A balanced diet rich in calcium, vitamin D, and other essential nutrients supports bone density. Foods such as dairy products, leafy greens, and fortified cereals should be included in daily meals to provide the necessary nutrients for maintaining strong bones.

However, dietary changes should be combined with other lifestyle factors, such as regular exercise and avoiding smoking or excessive alcohol consumption, for optimal prevention. A multifaceted approach is crucial for effectively managing bone health.

Is Exercise Too Risky for People with Osteoporosis?

Exercise is not too risky for individuals with osteoporosis; in fact, it is beneficial and crucial for maintaining bone density. Low-impact weight-bearing activities, such as walking, dancing, and resistance training, can help strengthen bones and improve balance, reducing the risk of falls and fractures. It's essential to consult with a healthcare professional to develop a safe and effective exercise plan tailored to individual needs.

Those with osteoporosis should avoid high-impact activities and exercises that increase the risk of falls. Instead, focusing on balance, flexibility, and strength training can provide significant benefits while minimizing injury risk.

Do Fractures Heal Completely in People with Osteoporosis?

Fractures in people with osteoporosis may not heal completely or as quickly as in those with healthy bone density. The healing process can be complicated by weakened bones, which increases the likelihood of future fractures. It's essential for individuals with osteoporosis to follow their healthcare provider's guidance during recovery to ensure optimal healing.

After a fracture, rehabilitation exercises and physical therapy can play a crucial role in regaining strength and mobility. Adhering to a prescribed recovery plan will help maximize healing and prevent further complications.

Is Osteoporosis Only a Concern After Menopause?

While osteoporosis is often associated with postmenopausal women due to decreased estrogen levels, it can affect individuals of all ages. Factors such as family history, lifestyle choices, and certain medical conditions can contribute to osteoporosis risk. Awareness and prevention efforts should begin earlier in life to mitigate future risks.

Both men and women should monitor their bone health throughout their lives, with regular bone density screenings starting around age 50 or earlier for those at risk. Understanding that osteoporosis is a broader concern can encourage proactive health management.

Can Osteoporosis Be Reversed with Treatment?

Osteoporosis can be managed effectively with various treatments, but it may not be completely reversible. Medications such as bisphosphonates, hormone replacement therapy, and newer drugs like monoclonal antibodies can help increase bone density and reduce fracture risk. It's vital to work closely with a healthcare provider to determine the most appropriate treatment plan.

In addition to medication, lifestyle changes like diet and exercise can significantly improve bone health.

Implementing these changes can lead to better outcomes in bone density and overall health.

Are Supplements Enough to Protect Bones?

While supplements like calcium and vitamin D can support bone health, they are not enough on their own to prevent osteoporosis. A well-rounded approach that includes a healthy diet, regular exercise, and lifestyle modifications is essential for maintaining strong bones. Supplements should be viewed as a complement to a healthy lifestyle rather than a sole solution.

Individuals should consult with a healthcare professional before starting any supplementation regimen to ensure they are meeting their specific nutritional needs. A comprehensive strategy is vital for effective osteoporosis management.

Is Bone Loss Always Noticeable?

Bone loss is often a silent process, meaning it can occur without noticeable symptoms until a fracture happens. Many people may not realize they have osteoporosis until they experience a broken bone from a minor fall or injury. Regular bone density screenings can help detect bone loss early, allowing for timely intervention.

To stay proactive about bone health, individuals should discuss screening options with their healthcare provider, especially if they have risk factors for osteoporosis. Being aware of one's bone health status is essential for preventing serious complications.

Can Osteoporosis Medications Harm Other Parts of the Body?

Some osteoporosis medications can have side effects that may impact other parts of the body. For example, bisphosphonates can occasionally cause gastrointestinal issues, and hormone therapies can increase the risk of blood clots. It's crucial to discuss potential risks and benefits with a healthcare provider when considering treatment options.

Monitoring health closely while on osteoporosis medications is essential. Regular check-ups and open communication with healthcare providers will help manage any side effects and ensure the treatment remains effective and safe.

Is Weight Training Safe for Osteoporosis Patients?

Weight training can be safe and beneficial for patients with osteoporosis, provided it is done correctly. Resistance exercises help improve bone density and strengthen muscles, which can enhance balance and reduce the risk of falls. Consulting with a healthcare provider or a trained physical therapist can ensure that exercises are appropriate for the individual's level of bone density.

When engaging in weight training, it's important to focus on proper form and start with light weights to avoid injury. Gradually increasing intensity while paying attention to body signals can lead to improved bone health and overall physical fitness.

Does Being Active Mean You Won't Get Osteoporosis?

While being physically active can significantly reduce the risk of osteoporosis, it does not guarantee immunity from the condition. Regular exercise, especially weight-bearing and resistance training, helps maintain bone density and overall health. However, other factors such as genetics, diet, and lifestyle also contribute to osteoporosis risk.

To enhance bone health, it's essential to incorporate a balanced lifestyle that includes regular exercise, a nutritious diet, and preventive healthcare measures. Combining these elements will help create a robust defense against osteoporosis.

Can Young People Develop Osteoporosis?

Yes, young people can develop osteoporosis, especially if they have risk factors such as a family history of the condition, low calcium intake, or certain medical conditions. Conditions like eating disorders or hormonal imbalances can also contribute to early bone density loss. Awareness is key to prevention and early intervention.

To promote healthy bone development in young people, it is crucial to encourage a balanced diet rich in calcium and vitamin D, as well as regular physical activity. Establishing healthy habits early on can help reduce the risk of osteoporosis later in life.

CHAPTER 9:

Frequently Asked Questions (FAQs)

What is the best test for diagnosing osteoporosis?

The best test for diagnosing osteoporosis is the Dual-Energy X-ray Absorptiometry (DXA) scan. This test measures bone mineral density (BMD) at key areas such as the hip and spine, helping to determine the risk of fractures. The DXA scan is non-invasive, involves minimal radiation exposure, and provides precise measurements that can guide treatment decisions.

For those concerned about their bone health, consult a healthcare provider to schedule a DXA scan. It's important to understand that a lower BMD score indicates a higher risk of osteoporosis, enabling you to take preventive actions early. This test is generally painless and takes only about 10-20 minutes to complete.

At what age should I start getting tested for bone density?

Women should generally start getting tested for bone density at age 65, while men should begin at age 70. However, if you have risk factors such as a family history of osteoporosis, previous fractures, or long-term use of medications like corticosteroids, your doctor may recommend testing earlier.

To get tested, speak with your healthcare provider about your personal risk factors and determine the right timeline for you. Regular testing helps track changes in bone density and assess the effectiveness of any treatment or lifestyle changes.

How much calcium and Vitamin D do I need daily?

Adults aged 19 to 50 should aim for 1,000 mg of calcium per day, while those over 50 need 1,200 mg. Vitamin D is essential for calcium absorption, with recommendations ranging from 600 IU (15 mcg) for those under 70, to 800 IU (20 mcg) for those over 70.

To meet these needs, incorporate calcium-rich foods like dairy products, leafy greens, and fortified foods into your diet. For Vitamin D, sun exposure, fatty fish, and fortified foods can help. If dietary sources are insufficient, consider supplements after consulting your healthcare provider.

Can I build back bone once it's lost?

While bone density can decrease with age and osteoporosis, it is possible to regain some bone mass through lifestyle changes. Engaging in weight-bearing exercises like walking, jogging, or resistance training can stimulate bone formation. A well-balanced diet rich in calcium and Vitamin D is also critical to support bone health.

Additionally, medical treatments such as bisphosphonates or hormone therapy may help build bone density. Speak with your healthcare provider to assess your situation and develop a comprehensive plan that includes exercise, diet, and potential medication.

What are the side effects of osteoporosis medications?

Osteoporosis medications, such as bisphosphonates, can cause side effects like gastrointestinal issues, flu-like symptoms, or jaw problems in rare cases. Other medications may lead to different side effects, so it's essential to discuss these with your doctor before starting treatment.

To minimize side effects, take medications as prescribed and maintain regular follow-up appointments with your healthcare provider. If you experience significant side effects, don't hesitate to report them, as your doctor can adjust your treatment plan or suggest alternatives.

How often should I get a bone density test?

The frequency of bone density tests can vary based on individual risk factors and initial results. Generally, if your results indicate normal bone density, testing every 2-3 years is sufficient. However, if you have low bone density or are undergoing treatment, your doctor may recommend annual testing to monitor progress.

It's crucial to follow your healthcare provider's advice regarding test intervals. Keeping track of your bone density over time allows for timely interventions if your bone health declines.

Are men at risk for osteoporosis?

Yes, men can develop osteoporosis, particularly after age 70 or if they have risk factors such as low testosterone levels, a family history of osteoporosis, or long-term steroid use. While women are at greater risk, osteoporosis in men can lead to significant fractures and health issues.

To address this risk, men should focus on maintaining a healthy lifestyle that includes adequate calcium and Vitamin D intake, regular exercise, and avoiding smoking or excessive alcohol consumption. Consulting with a healthcare provider can help assess individual risk and guide prevention strategies.

What type of doctor treats osteoporosis?

An endocrinologist or a rheumatologist is typically best suited to treat osteoporosis, as they specialize in hormonal and bone health issues. However, primary care physicians can also diagnose and manage osteoporosis, often collaborating with specialists for comprehensive care.

When seeking treatment, be prepared to discuss your medical history and undergo necessary tests. Your healthcare provider will develop a tailored treatment plan, which may include medication, lifestyle modifications, and regular monitoring of your bone health.

Is osteoporosis painful?

Osteoporosis itself is not painful; however, the fractures resulting from weakened bones can be extremely painful. Many individuals may not realize they have osteoporosis until they experience a fracture, often in the hip, spine, or wrist.

To manage pain associated with fractures, effective treatments may include pain relievers, physical therapy, and sometimes surgical interventions.

Early detection and treatment of osteoporosis can help reduce the risk of painful fractures.

How do I know if my exercise routine is helping my bones?

To determine if your exercise routine is benefiting your bone health, monitor your overall strength, balance, and mobility. Engaging in weight-bearing and resistance exercises can enhance bone density over time. You may notice improvements in your physical abilities, such as increased strength or stability, which are positive indicators.

Keep a record of your exercise routine and any changes in your physical condition. Regular consultations with a healthcare provider or physical therapist can also provide insight into your progress and necessary adjustments to your exercise plan.

Can children develop osteoporosis?

Yes, children can develop osteoporosis, often as a result of certain medical conditions, nutritional deficiencies, or lack of physical activity. Although rare, it is essential for children to have a healthy diet rich in calcium and Vitamin D, along with regular exercise, to build strong bones.

Parents should encourage healthy habits from an early age, including participating in weight-bearing activities and ensuring adequate nutrient intake. If there are concerns about a child's bone health, consulting a pediatrician or specialist can help identify potential issues and guide appropriate interventions.

How long will I need to take osteoporosis medication?

The duration of osteoporosis medication can vary based on individual factors such as bone density results, age, and overall health. Some individuals may require treatment for several years, while others may only need it for a shorter period.

Regular follow-up appointments and bone density tests will help your healthcare provider determine the effectiveness of the medication and whether adjustments are needed. Always discuss any concerns about long-term medication use with your doctor, as they can provide guidance tailored to your specific situation.

Can diet alone manage osteoporosis?

While a balanced diet is crucial for managing osteoporosis, it may not be sufficient on its own. A diet rich in calcium, Vitamin D, and other essential nutrients supports bone health, but physical activity and medical treatments are also vital components of osteoporosis management.

To effectively manage osteoporosis, combine a healthy diet with weight-bearing exercises and, if necessary, medications prescribed by a healthcare provider. This comprehensive approach can help optimize bone health and reduce the risk of fractures.

Conclusion

o prevent and manage osteoporosis effectively, focus on a balanced diet rich in calcium and vitamin D. Incorporate foods like dairy products, leafy greens, and fortified cereals into your meals. It's also essential to engage in weight-bearing exercises, such as walking or resistance training, which help strengthen bones and improve balance.

Regular screenings for bone density are crucial, especially for those at risk. Medications may be necessary for some individuals, so working with a healthcare provider to develop a personalized plan is key. Staying informed about osteoporosis can empower individuals to take control of their bone health.

Printed in Great Britain
by Amazon

8a54e1e2-8793-461d-b2e9-4944807a7edaR01